Gravity and the Circulation

The Principle of Hydrocaptivity

James Munis, MD, PhD

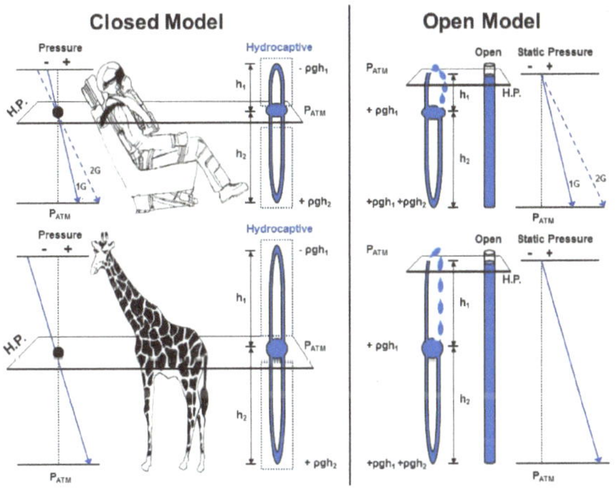

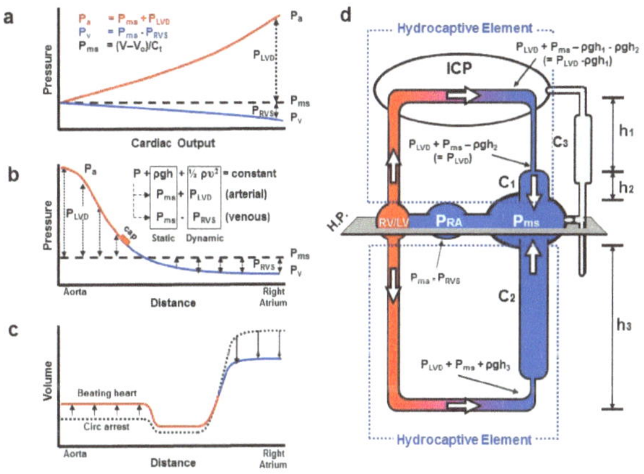

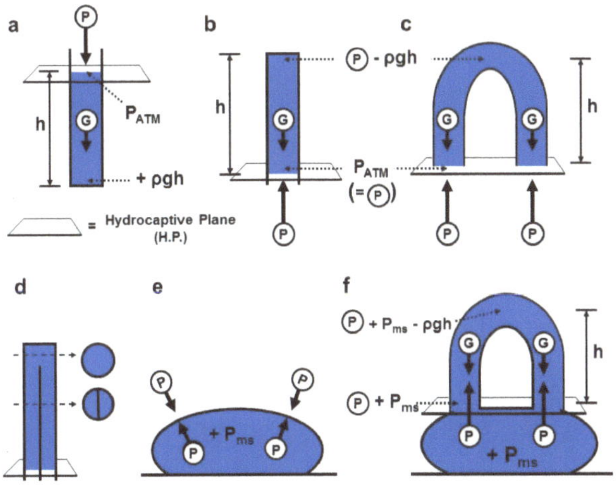

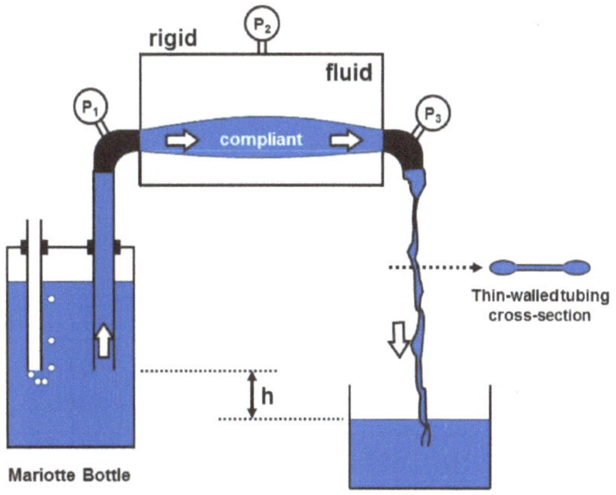

Context and History

As blood circulates through the systemic circulation, it is subject to three forces, each of which contributes to a composite pressure profile. This profile changes along the course of the circulation, but returns to its original value at the completion of the circuit. The individual components of pressure derive from: 1) atmospheric, 2) hydrostatic, and 3) vascular or cardiac wall sources. The latter can, in turn, derive from active smooth muscle contraction, passive elastic recoil, or passive transmission of tissue pressures through the vessel wall.

Over the course of more than three centuries, a number of physical principles and physiological observations have been applied to the mammalian circulation, where, in aggregate, they have begun to complete a picture of the cardiovascular system as a single hydraulic entity. These include William Harvey's description of the cardiovascular system as a complete and closed system (21), Pascal's Principle of hydrostatic pressure and its transmission throughout a fluid continuum (19), Newton's Laws of Motion, Bernoulli's Principle of total fluid energy for a fluid in motion, and the Hagen-Poiseuille Law for laminar flow (14).

As our ability to describe the hydraulics of individual components of the system has matured, however, many commonly used conceptual models have strayed from Harvey's first observation that the cardiovascular system is a complete and closed circuit. This tendency may have arisen from an effort to avoid the complexity that arises from including gravitational and postural considerations, as well as difficulties that arise from closed-loop, rather than segmental, fluid dynamics. For example, the representation of the human cerebral circulation in its usual upright posture necessitates the inclusion of closed-system hydraulics – a topic that may be counterintuitive or confusing. Similarly, the representation of "venous return curves" may attempt avoid the difficulties inherent in a closed system model by instead dividing the closed loop of the systemic circulation into a segment bounded at one end by mean systemic pressure, and at the other end, by right atrial pressure. However, this segmental analysis can, and has, led to confusion and controversy about circulatory hydraulics (5, 6, 35). Similarly, the representation of left ventricular pressure-volume loops may give an adequate picture of isolated left ventricular mechanics, but it does so at the expense of neglecting the rest of the circuit and the interdependence of its individual components.

As humans have ventured into the weightless environment of space and low earth orbit, as well as into the multiple G-force acceleration environments of aerospace, and as physiological studies have included the extraordinary phenomenon seen in comparative physiology, including cerebral blood flow in the giraffe, the lack of a common-use model of the cardiovascular system that can accommodate these differential force environments, species, and postural changes becomes evident.

The model presented here is built stepwise, keeping in mind the functional requirement that it must be robust enough to accommodate the features listed above, particularly those resulting from changes in gravity and posture, as well as represent a complete and closed circuit. It also takes into account that many vascular conduits are partially collapsible. For the more counterintuitive or controversial elements (for example, flow through vertically oriented collapsible conduit and flow through collapsible conduit contained within a relatively isovolemic cranium), data from a physical model are presented in order to validate the conceptual model.

Step 1. The concept of "Hydrocaptivity"

The combined effects of gravity-related fluid (hydrostatic) pressure and atmospheric pressure (P_{ATM}) are represented in Figure 1. At the surface of the Earth, the hydrostatic pressure derived from gravitational force is oriented downward, and depicted as a vector labeled "G". P_{ATM} is depicted as a vector labeled "P".

It is important to note that P_{ATM} has no directional component within the small dimensions of the cardiovascular system; but rather, acts simultaneously in all directions. Nonetheless, when a fluid is contained within a boundary that insulates some of its surfaces, but not others, from P$_{ATM}$, the effect of P$_{ATM}$ now has a directional component – acting only at, and normal to, the exposed surface of the contained fluid. I will refer to this directional effect of P$_{ATM}$ on a partially contained fluid as "hydrocaptivity" since it may result in the confinement of the fluid within its open container even when the opening faces downward. This same effect is evident when fluid is retained within a vertical drinking straw when a finger seals the upper end.

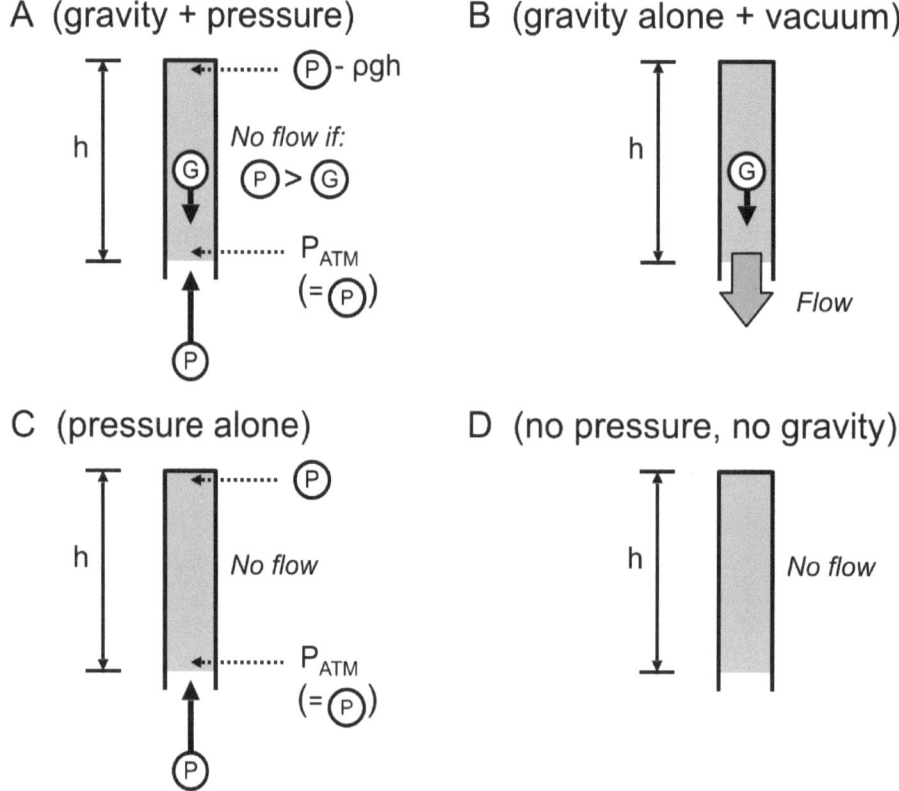

Figure 1. The concept of "Hydrocaptivity"

In the case of Fig. 1A, fluid within a vertically-oriented container is exposed to a downward-directed hydrostatic pressure ("G") and also to an oppositely-directed atmospheric pressure ("P"). The resulting force vectors summate. If P$_{ATM}$ > G (quantitatively, G = ρgh, where ρ = density of fluid; g = acceleration due to gravity, and h = height above a reference level), the fluid will remain within the container and no outward flow will occur. At the opening of the container, the pressure of the fluid = P_{ATM}. At the top of the container, it is = $P_{ATM} - \rho gh$.

Fig.1B represents the same fluid-filled container exposed to 1g at the surface of the Earth, but in a vacuum with no exposure to P_{ATM}. Without the opposing effect of P_{ATM}, fluid will flow out of the container under the influence of gravity.

Fig. 1C represents the same system exposed to P_{ATM} alone without exposure to a gravitational vector, as might occur in a spacecraft pressurized to 1 ATM in a weightless orbital environment. Because the fluid is exposed to P_{ATM} alone without the opposing force of gravity, no flow out of the container occurs. Furthermore, there is no pressure gradient within the fluid since $\rho gh = 0$ throughout its vertical extent. Absent an effect of gravity, the fluid simply acts to transmit atmospheric pressure throughout its continuum at all heights. Pascal's principle does not apply in the normal sense of having the qualification that pressure is equally distributed through the fluid continuum at the same height since height is irrelevant in this gravity-free circumstance.

Fig. 1D represents the same system in the absence of either gravity or atmospheric pressure, as might occur in the weightlessness and vacuum of space. No flow will occur out of the container, and no pressure gradients will occur within the fluid.

Step 2: The application of a "hydrocaptive plane"

Figure 2 confines all observations to a 1G force environment at the surface of the Earth, and to a normal sea-level P_{ATM}. This step considers the effect of orientation in space on the pressure profile within a partially contained fluid. It then applies the same analysis to the case of an inverted U tube, open at both ends. Finally, it considers the joining of an inverted U tube to an elastic, fluid-filled container. A plane is defined as a "hydrocaptive plane" ("H.P."). This is in contrast to a hydrostatic indifference "point" because it encompasses, simultaneously, two openings which occur at the same vertical level within the same fluid continuity.

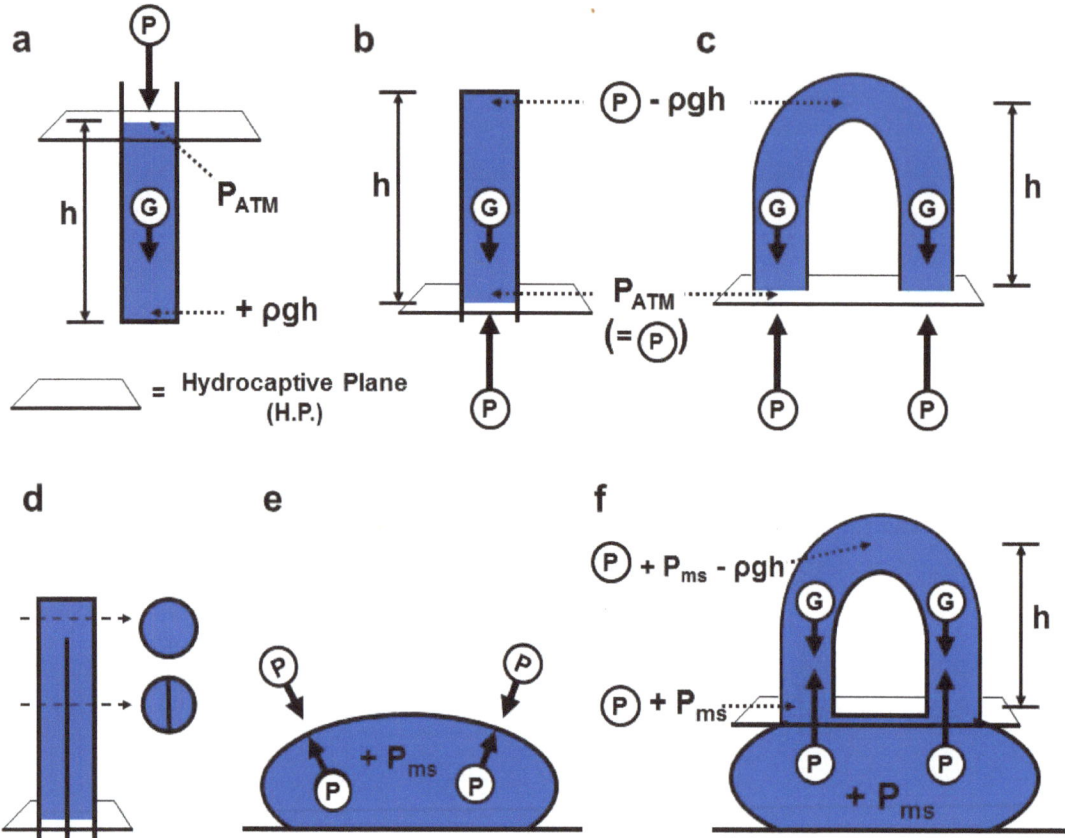

Figure 2. The application of a "hydrocaptive plane"

Fig. 2A An upright, fluid –filled cylinder open at the top. P_{ATM} acts in a downward direction only because of the orientation of the opening. G acts in the same, downward, orientation to summate with P_{ATM}.

Pressure at the surface = P_{ATM}. Pressure at the bottom = ρgh, where h = height of fluid column. A hydrocaptive plane (H.P.) occurs at the interface between the fluid and air. At the H.P., the fluid pressure will remain the same (P_{ATM}) even if the container is inverted (as in Fig. 1A) as long as $\rho gh < P_{ATM}$.

Fig. 2B The case of inverting the container in 2A. Pressure at the H.P. = P_{ATM}. Pressure at the (now inverted) top of the container = $- \rho gh$. The H.P. remains at the level of the air-fluid interface.

Figs. 2C and 2D Considers a bisecting membrane extending part way up the inverted container of 2B (cross-sections shown in 2D). The presence of this membrane does not change the vertical hydraulic profile or the position of the H.P. within the container. The two sides of the bisected cylinder are now separated and reshaped to form an inverted U tube. The same hydraulic profile pertains, as does the position of the H.P.

Fig. 2E The case of a fluid-filled, elastic container resting on a solid surface. The pressure within the container is defined as P_{ms} ("mean systemic pressure"), which is the physiologic equivalent of $V-V_0/C$, where V = total fluid (or blood) volume; V_0 = unstressed volume; and C = compliance. Within this step of the model, vertical pressure gradients within the container are not considered, as they will be added in subsequent steps. P_{ATM} acts at all container-air interfaces, and P_{ATM} summates with Pms to distribute evenly within the fluid continuum according to Pascal's principle. Note that P_{ATM} contributes to the absolute pressure within the elastic container, but does not change the transmural pressure across the walls of the container since it acts equally on both sides.

Fig. 2F Joining of the containers in 2C and 2E. The H.P. remains at the interface between the rigid inverted U tube and the adjacent area of compliance – in this case, at the top of the elastic container. Because the pressure within the elastic container = P_{ms}, the pressure at the H.P. is also P_{ms}.

Step 3: The application of mean systemic pressure (Pms) and the addition of a "cranial" component that contains collapsible conduit within a fluid-filled, isovolemic system.

Fig. 3A Defines stressed and unstressed blood volume. Pressure is measured as fluid is infused into an empty elastic container. No pressure increase occurs until "unstressed volume" (V_0) is reached. Volume infused above V_0 contributes to a pressure increase along an elastance curve. This additional volume that contributes to pressure is referred to as "stressed blood volume", and is defined as the difference between total volume and stressed volume ($V - V_0$).

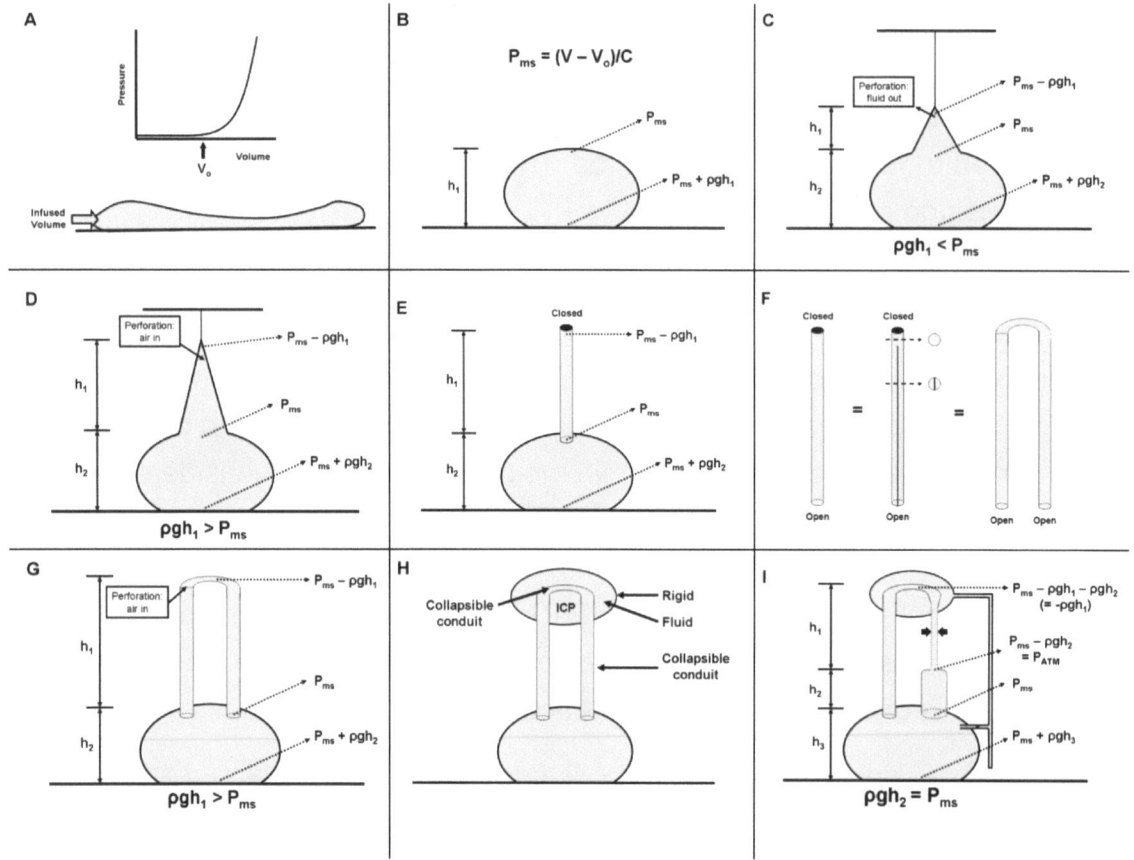

Figure 3. The application of mean systemic pressure (Pms) and the addition of a "cranial" component that contains collapsible conduit within a fluid-filled, isovolemic system

Fig. 3B Defines mean systemic pressure (P_{ms}). P_{ms} = stressed volume/compliance = $(V − V_0)/C$. Within the confines of the elastic container, a vertical hydrostatic gradient (ρgh) summates with P_{ms}.

Fig. 3C Considers the partial suspension of the compliant fluid-filled container from a single point from above. Wall tension in the upper portion increases, and along with it, elastance. The boundary between the more stretched (less compliant) wall above and the more compliant wall below is demarcated as the boundary between h1 and h2, respectively. The volume contained within the region h1 is considered "hydrocaptive" and is at least partially insulated from PATM. This allows for the presence of sub-Pms pressure above the h1 – h2 boundary. Pressure within the container as a whole follows a vertical hydrostatic gradient as indicated. Because $\rho gh1 < P_{ms}$, a theoretical perforation in the upper portion of the container will result in fluid leaking out, rather than air leaking in.

Fig. 3D A similar system as in 3C, except the container is suspended more from above and supported less by the surface below. In this case, the portion of the container that is stretched (and therefore, rigid enough to be hydrocaptive) is greater than in 3C. Because $\rho gh1 > P_{ms}$, subatmospheric pressure occurs in the upper reaches of the stretched (hydrocaptive) portion of the container. At the indicated point of a theoretical perforation, air would leak in, rather than fluid leak out.

Fig. 3E A fluid-filled, rigid cylinder now replaces the stretched, or hydrocaptive, part of 3D. Whether or not sub-atmospheric pressure is achieved within the cylinder depends on the relative magnitude of $\rho gh1$ and P_{ms}. If $\rho gh1 > P_{ms}$, sub-atmospheric pressure will result at the top of the cylinder. If $\rho gh1 < P_{ms}$, it will not. In either case, a hydrostatic pressure gradient will exist with all pressures above the boundary between the rigid cylinder and the elastic container will be less than Pms.

Fig. 3F A reiteration of Fig 2D demonstrating the equivalence of an inverted U tube to the an inverted cylinder.

Fig. 3G Replacing the inverted cylinder in 3E with an inverted U tube. The inverted U tube now constitutes the hydrocaptive element of the system, and the hydrostatic pressures within are as indicated.

Fig. 3H The upper portion of the rigid inverted U tube is replaced with compliant tubing. This portion of the U tube is, in turn, encompassed within a rigid, fluid-filled shell. Because this shell and its contents constitute an isovolumic system with non-expansible fluid contents, the filled compliant tubing cannot collapse (see Fig. 6 for specific demonstration of this principle). One vertical limb of the inverted U tube is also replaced with compliant tubing (jugular vein).

Fig. 3I System depicted in 3H after pressure equilibration. An additional element representing the cerebrospinal fluid (CSF) buffer is represented, along with a variably-adjustable valve at the connection between CSF and blood volumes. Note the differential transmural pressures within the vertical compliant tubing. In the lower aspect of the vertical tubing, transmural pressure is positive and the compliant vertical tubing bulges outward. At the transition point where $\rho gh = P_{ms}$, the pressure within the tubing = P_{ATM}. Above that point, pressure is subatmospheric and the tubing tends to collapse. Pressures in the opposite vertical (rigid) element are the same as within the compliant tubing at any level, in adherence with Pascal's principle.

Step 4: Effects of varying gravitational acceleration (+Gz) on a combined hydrocaptive/compliant system.

Fig. 4A Comparison of the pressure profile behavior between two systems: a fluid-filled rigid inverted U tube joined to a fluid-filled elastic container, versus a fluid-filled cylinder open at the top, when subjected to increased downward (+Gz) gravitational acceleration. The perforations depicted in the cylinder demonstrate the relative tendency of fluid to leak out at vertical levels. Note the qualitatively different behaviors between the two systems, including the presence of subatmospheric pressure within the inverted U tube/elastic container and the absence of subatmospheric pressure in the cylinder. A H.P. exists at the air-fluid interface of the cylinder and at the interface between the hydrocaptive element and the compliant body of the opposite system. At the H.P., pressure is independent of +Gz forces.

Fig. 4B Same system as in 4A, except that behavior of the cylinder is depicted only at points below the air-fluid interface.

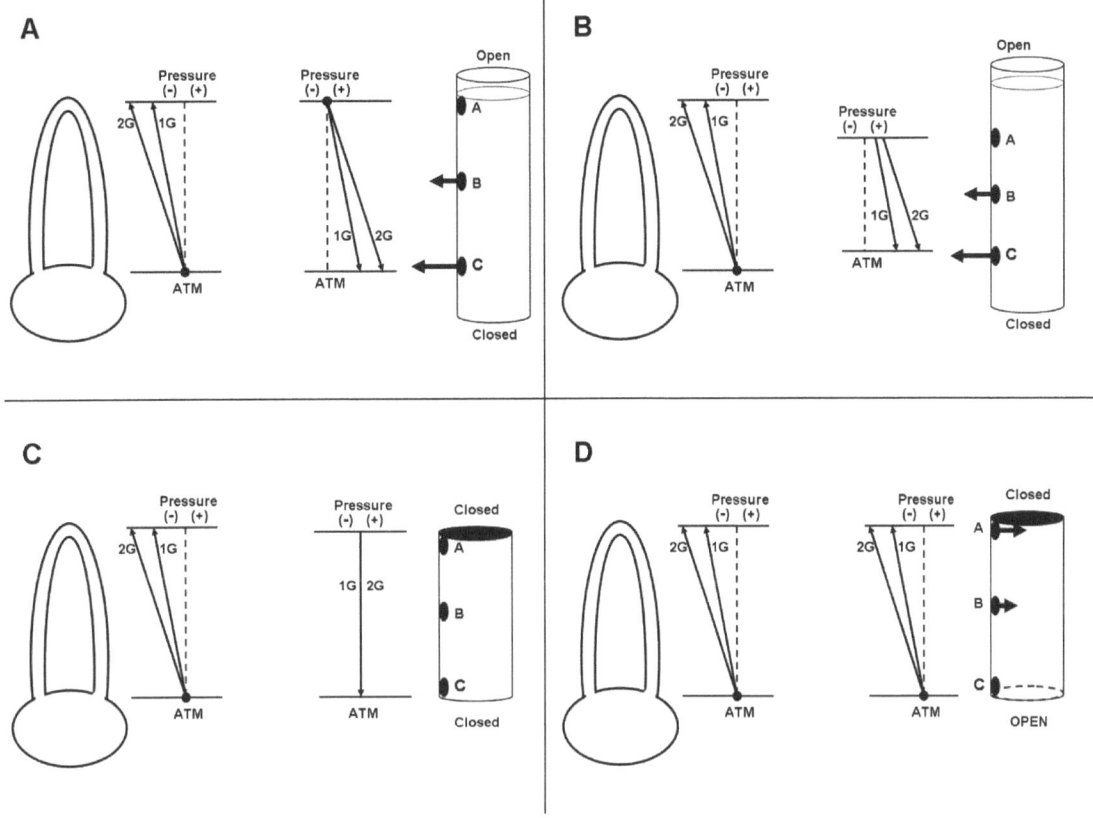

Figure 4. Effects of varying gravitational acceleration (+Gz) on a combined hydrocaptive/compliant system

Fig. 4C Same comparison, but with a rigid fluid-filled cylinder closed at both ends.

Fig. 4D Same comparison, but with an inverted cylinder open only at the bottom. In this case, the inverted cylinder constitutes a hydrocaptive element. Theoretical perforations indicate the relative tendency of air moving into the cylinder at different vertical levels. A H.P. exists at the air-fluid interface of the cylinder.

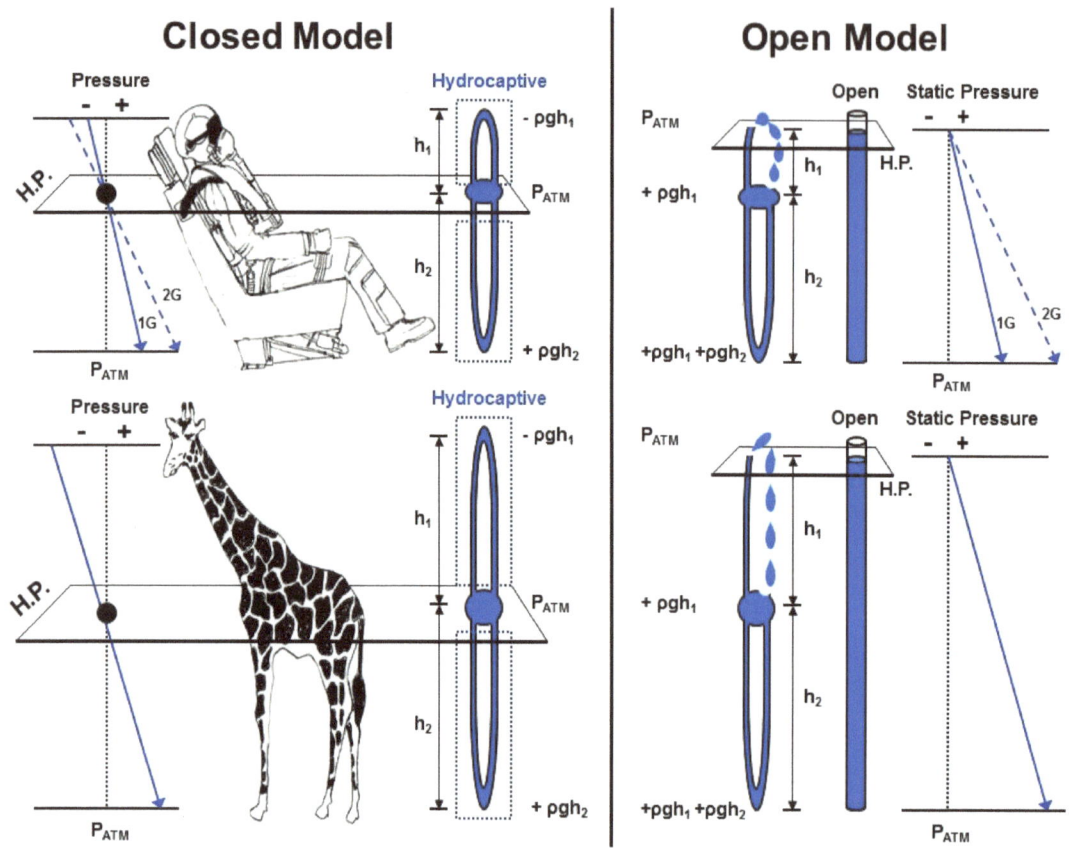

Figure 5. Comparing the behavior of open vs. closed (hydrocaptive) systems under varying +Gz acceleration.

Step 5: Comparing the behaviors of open vs closed (hydrocaptive) systems under varying +Gz acceleration.

The hydrocaptive model, but not the open model, mimics the behavior of the human circulation under varying +Gz, as well as the vertical pressure profile of the standing giraffe. In this depiction, the open model is represented both as a cylinder of fluid open at the top, or as a compliant center chamber connected to a downward recurrent circulatory loop and to an open upwardly-directed conduit that empties into the air with a "waterfall" venous return. For clarity, cardiac-generated pressures are not included in this schematic, so it represents hydrostatic and atmospheric pressures alone. The hydrocaptive, or closed, model contains both an upwardly and downwardly-directed circulatory loop, joined at a compliant middle chamber and lacking any open-air or waterfall feature. The two rigid circulatory loops each constitute a hydrocaptive element. A H.P. exists at the level of the compliant middle chamber – coinciding with the heart-level of both the astronaut and the giraffe. Experimental data from aerospace physiology studies (see Wood et al.) indicate that vascular pressure at heart level remains constant, while pressures above the heart fall and below the heart rise, as a function of increasing +Gz acceleration. This is predicted by the closed, hydrocaptive model, but not by either open model. Data from the standing giraffe indicate a H.P. located at heart level, not head level, even though there is fluid continuity from head to foot within the arterial system. This is also predicted by the closed, hydrocaptive model but not by either open model.

Step 6: Demonstration of the inability of an elastic body to collapse when contained within a rigid, isovolemic, fluid-filled enclosure.

This physical model demonstrates the principle of why otherwise "collapsible" veins or sinuses may not collapse within the confines of a fluid-filled, rigid, enclosure like the cranium.

Fig. 6A An air-filled elastic balloon is attached to the inside opening of an air/water-tight spigot of an air-tight glass container. The spigot is closed and the balloon remains inflated. The container is filled with water, displacing all air outside of the inflated balloon. The top of the container is sealed, with the air/water-tight valve on the top of the container closed. A "balloon-shaped" air space now remains within the container, surrounded by water.

Fig. 6B The same system as in 6A, but inverted. The balloon has a tendency to move upward, but remains inflated, as before.

Fig. 6C The same system as in 6A, but with the spigot opened to atmosphere. The balloon inside the container, which is now inn communication with the atmosphere, remains inflated.

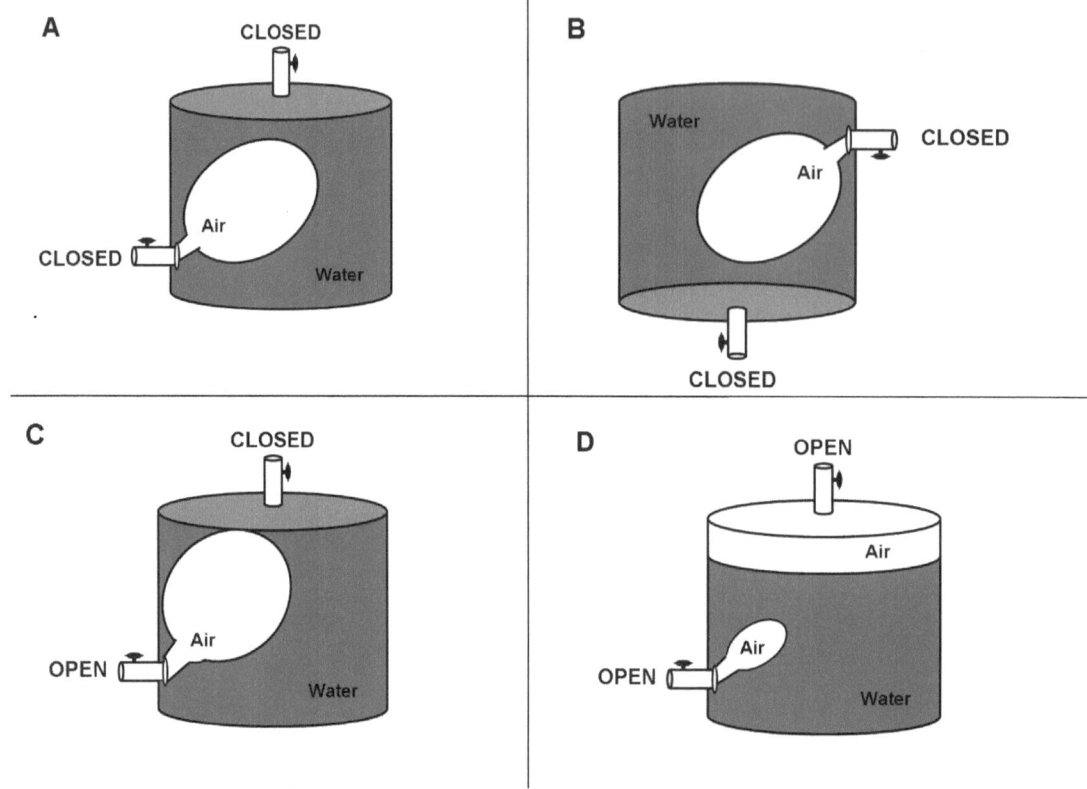

Figure 6. Demonstration of the inability of an elastic body to collapse when contained within a rigid, isovolemic, fluid-filled enclosure

Fig. 6D The valve on the top is now opened, allowing atmospheric air to displace water, which can, in turn, now displace the air escaping from the balloon and out through the spigot.

Steps 7 and 8: A physical model of the cerebral circulation, containing compliant conduit within a fluid-filled, rigid, isovolemic, cranium as well as a compliant vertical conduit mimicking the jugular venous system. The model is observed to support continuous fluid flow without resorting to a positive pressure source, and sustains subatmospheric pressure within the cranial component. By substituting a siphon flow source with unequal vertical limbs in place of a positive pressure (cardiac) pump, the model tests the hypothesis that a cranial-like circulation can maintain flow even through collapsible segments and even while subject to negative transmural pressure.

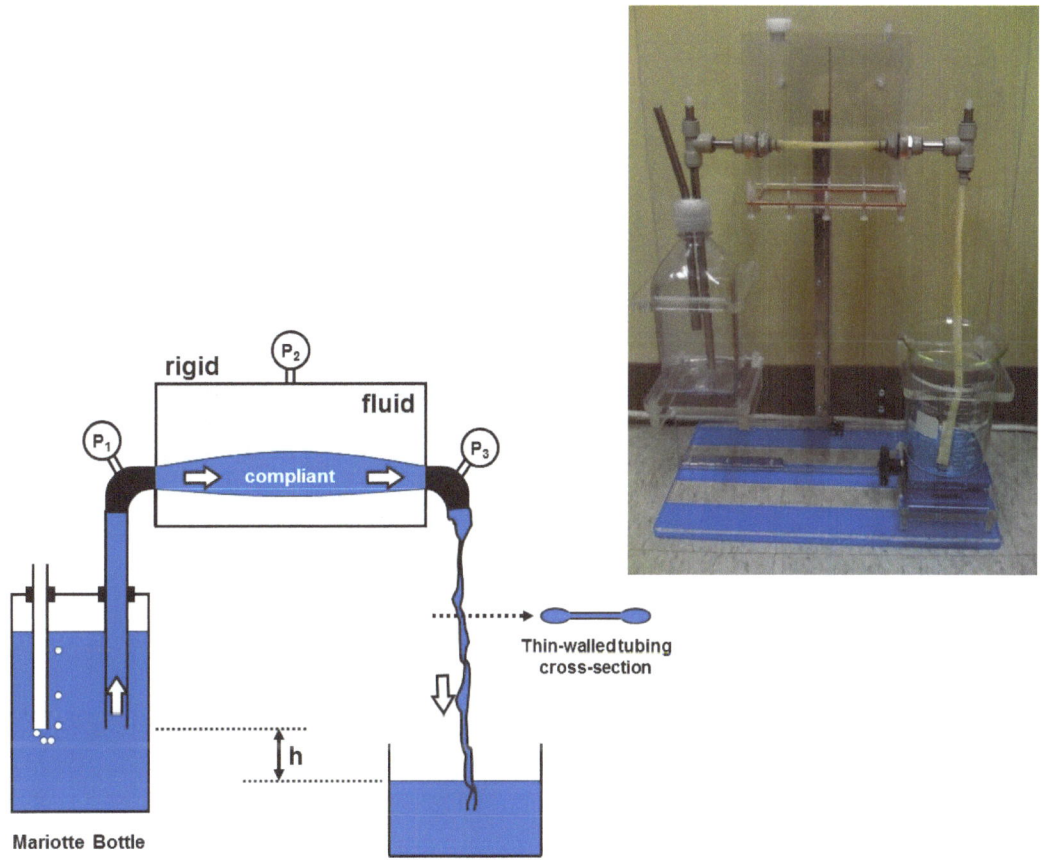

Figure 7. A physical model of the cerebral circulation, containing compliant conduit within a fluid-filled, rigid, isovolemic, cranium as well as a compliant vertical conduit mimicking the jugular venous system

Fig. 7 This model was constructed with plexiglass walls and air-tight joints and fittings (Mayo Clinic Rochester, Division of Engineering), using ¼ inch / 6.35 mm I.D. Penrose drains (Bard, Covington, GA) for both the compliant portion of the intracranial circulation and for the jugular circulation. The dimensions of the "cranial" enclosure were 15 x 15 x 6 cm (h, w, d), with a 25 cm total vertical distance between the inlet port into the "cranial" enclosure and the bottom of the attached tubing within the Mariotte bottle. The inlet and outlet ports of the cranial enclosure were located 5 cm above the base of the enclosure. Flow was established with a siphon system, using a Mariotte bottle as the upper water bath and an open container as the lower bath. The Mariotte bottle was chosen for the upper water bath source since it maintains a constant hydrostatic pressure source even as the water level within the bottle falls (31). The lower water bath can be raised or lowered, as required, to alter perfusion pressure. Flow is calculated by stepwise volume/time ratios observed in the lower water bath. During flow, the vertical (jugular) Penrose drain was partially collapsed, but maintained patency and fluid continuity in the open corners. During all flow conditions, the transmural pressure ("P") in the isovolumic container remained at -19 to -21 mmHg, as measured with an electronic strain gauge transducer (Edwards Lifesciences, Irvine, CA) and monitor (Hewlett-Packard Omnicare, Palo Alto, CA).

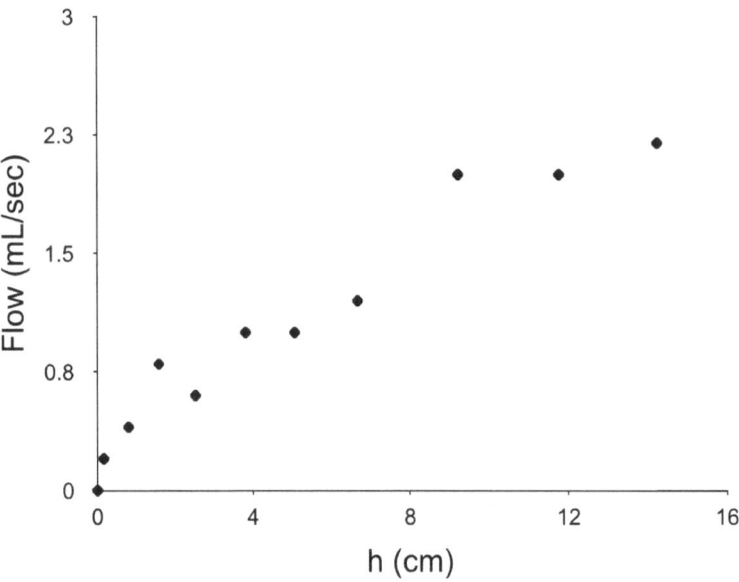

Figure 8. Hydrostatic gradient versus flow results

Fig. 8 Hydrostatic gradient versus flow results. At vertical gradient = 0, no flow occurred. As the vertical gradient was increased in a stepwise fashion, flow increased in an essentially linear manner. At no point during the experiment did the intracranial Penrose drain collapse – consistent with the observations in Fig. 6.

Step 9: Addition of a compliant component to the theoretical model, both above and below heart level, and behavior under increased +Gz.

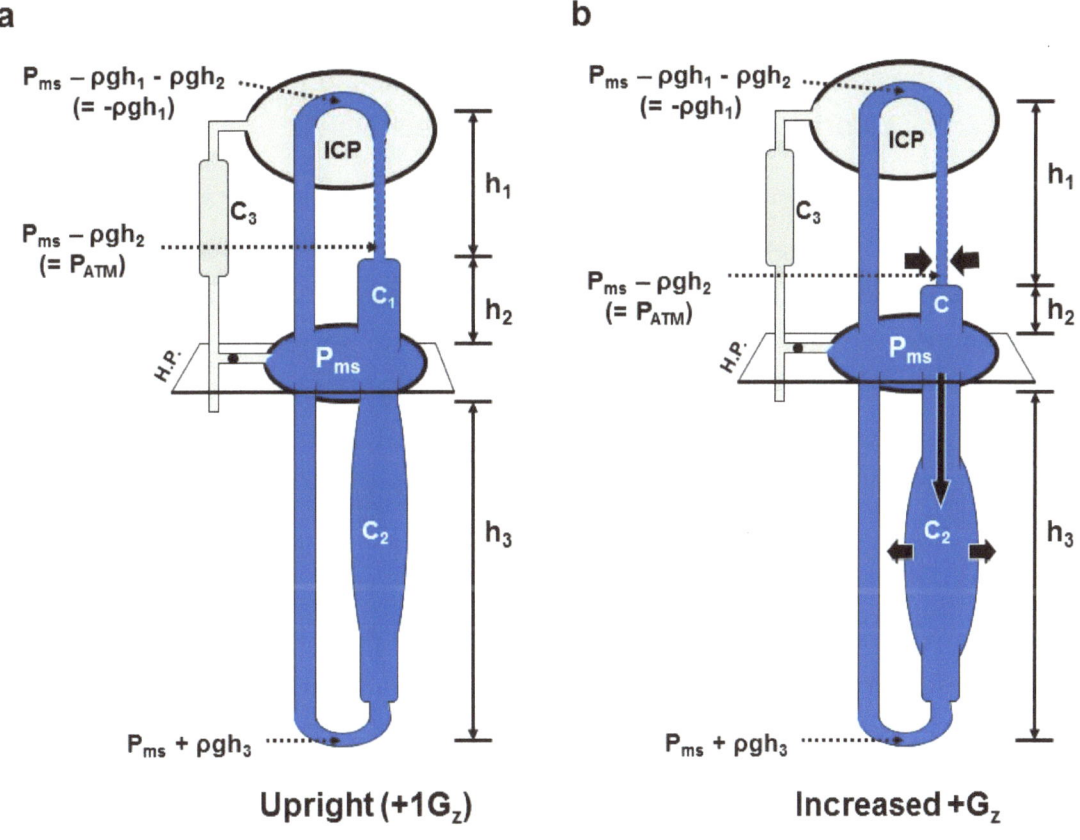

a

$P_{ms} - \rho gh_1 - \rho gh_2$
$(= -\rho gh_1)$

$P_{ms} - \rho gh_2$
$(= P_{ATM})$

$P_{ms} + \rho gh_3$

Upright (+1G$_z$)

b

$P_{ms} - \rho gh_1 - \rho gh_2$
$(= -\rho gh_1)$

$P_{ms} - \rho gh_2$
$(= P_{ATM})$

$P_{ms} + \rho gh_3$

Increased +G$_z$

Figure 9. Addition of a compliant component to the theoretical model, both above and below heart level, and behavior under increased +Gz

Fig. 9A The model now includes a compliant segment above heart-level (C1) and below heart-level (C2) in the equivalent of venous return reservoirs (approximating the jugular venous and inferior vena cava systems, respectively). The model is assumed to be in an upright position, and the H.P. occurs at heart-level. In the jugular system, the transition from positive to negative transmural pressure occurs at height h2 above heart-level, where $\rho gh2 = P_{ms}$. At this step, the model does not yet include a cardiac pressure source. Instead, it resolves atmospheric and hydrostatic pressure profiles alone, without a dynamic component. The cerebral portion of the circulation is contained within a rigid, fluid-filled, isovolemic cranium that surrounds compliant conduit. As demonstrated in Fig 6 and Fig 7, this "collapsible" conduit will not collapse within this enclosure. A CSF reservoir communicates with both the intracranial space (designated as "ICP" for "intracranial pressure"), as well as a vertical area of compliance (C3) representing the spinal subarachnoid space. The latter, in turn, communicates with the central blood compartment through a check-valve.

Fig. 9B The same model as 9A, but subject to increased +Gz acceleration. Some volume of blood will translocate from the upper to the lower compliant areas. Because h2 is now decreased (satisfying the requirement that $\rho gh2 = P_{ms}$ while g has increased), the transition point between positive and negative transmural pressure within the jugular system has moved downward, and a greater length of jugular vein will be in a partially collapsed state. In vivo, this will also result in an increased jugular venous and overall cerebrovascular resistance.

Step 10: Completion of the systemic circulation model to include a cardiac pressure and flow source.

Fig. 10D incorporates a combined right-ventricular and left-ventricular cardiac pump. The pulmonary circulation is not separately considered in this model. The upwardly-oriented and downwardly-oriented recurrent circulatory loops each constitute a partially hydrocaptive element. The designation as "partially" hydro-captive underscores that areas of compliance within a fluid-filled container or conduit do not insulate the contained fluid from P_{ATM}. The resulting pressure profile is displayed. "P_{LVD}" denotes "left-ventricular-derived" pressure; and "PRVS" denotes "right-ventricular-suction-derived" pressure. The former is addi

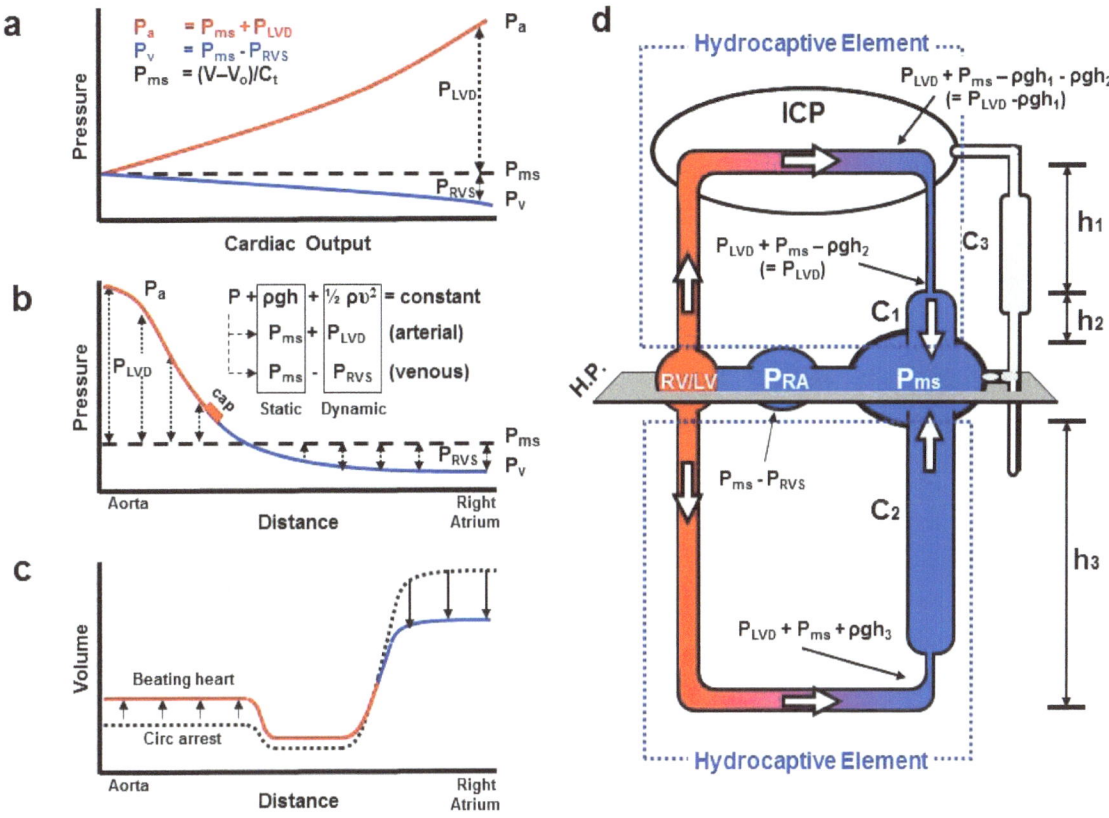

Figure 10. Completion of the systemic circulation model to include a cardiac pressure and flow source

tive to the static pressure profile and the latter is subtracted from the same profile. P_{LVD} and P_{RVS} add and subtract, respectively, pressure to or from P_{ms}.

Fig 10A Definitions of arterial (P_a), central venous (P_v), and mean systemic (circulatory arrest – P_{ms}) pressures, along with a graphical representation of vascular pressures as a function of cardiac-generated flow through a systemic resistance and superimposed on P_{ms}. This graphical representation is equivalent to both the theoretical and empirical results of Levy's analysis (Levy, 1979). It is also the abscissa-inverted equivalent of Starling's demonstration, using a model

19

of progressive acute cardiac tamponade (Starling, 1897), demonstrating arterial and central venous pressures as a function of progressively impaired cardiac output. The differential arterial and central venous pressure excursions from Pms are a consequence of differential arterial and central venous compliances.

Fig. 10B Graphical representation of the systemic pressure profile as a function of distance through the systemic circulation. At the same crossover point between systemic pressure and Pms noted by Starling (Starling, 1897), vascular pressure is independent of cardiac activity and has no dynamic component. Proximal to this point, vascular pressures are elevated above P_{ms} by P_{LVD}, which degrades through resistance; and below this point, vascular pressures are depressed below P_{ms} by P_{RVS}. As also first noted by Starling, the position of capillaries is proximal to this point. The first equation is that of Bernoulli, restating that total pressure, including both a static ($P + \rho gh$) and a dynamic ($1/2\ \rho u2$) component, remains constant after frictional heat loss is accounted for.

Fig. 10C Graphical representation of blood volume translocation as a function of distance through the systemic circulation, comparing cardiac arrest to functional circulation. As with 10A and 10B, this graphical analysis emphasizes that flow (cardiac output) is an independent variable, and pressure gradients are a dependent variable, or the result of pressure-volume work performed by the heart in translocating blood from venous to arterial compartments.

Implications

In 1628, Harvey demonstrated that the cardiovascular system is a closed loop (21). In 1647, Pascal, following on the ideas of Torricelli, demonstrated that the opposing forces of atmospheric and hydrostatic pressure reach equilibrium within recurrent loops, or siphons. Although Pascal never applied his analysis of siphon behaviour to the cardiovascular system, his findings held implications for resolving the relationship between gravity and blood flow in a closed-system conduit. In 1762, Bernoulli refined this understanding by including a gravitational force term when he applied the concept of conservation of energy to a description of both the static and dynamic components of pressure within a fluid continuum. In the twentieth century, Burton integrated much of this work by applying Pascal's hydrostatic concepts and the Bernoulli equation to an analysis of the circulation (8). Burton stopped short, however, of developing an integrated model of the systemic circulation that could predict hemodynamic responses to changes in the gravitational force environment or body posture.

The Principle of Hydrocaptivity

The concept of "hydrocaptivity", when applied to the sum of the systemic vascular loops, makes testable predictions about intravascular pressure profiles and their responses to gravity. It also predicts the position of a "hydrocaptive plane" within the circulation. The existence of this plane can be verified by a reexamination of measurements in altered force environments, such as those encountered in aerospace physiology experiments, with altered body positions, or in the terrestrial test case of the giraffe. In 1956, Guyton determined that a "physiologic reference point" exists within the mammalian circulation where pressure is insensitive to changes in body position, and therefore, to changes in the direction of the gravitational force vector (18, 26). The same concept was discussed a half century earlier by Hill, who referred to it as a "hydrostatic indifference point" (25). Guyton attributed the existence of this point to the servo-control of right atrial pressure by the Frank-Starling law of the heart, but he did not consider a simple hydrostatic explanation involving the principles first elucidated by Pascal and Bernoulli.

A fluid-filled container or conduit will demonstrate hydrocaptivity if it excludes air and if it is supported internally or externally. The conduit may communicate with a compliant element; or in the case of an inverted container, if it communicates at its downward opening with the atmosphere. Fluid within a hydrocaptive element will not fall out even when inverted as long as the balance of atmospheric and hydrostatic pressures favor its retention. Fig. 1 demonstrates a variety of both hydrocaptive and non-hydrocaptive elements, and the combination of the two, in the beginnings of the hemodynamic model shown in Fig. 1F. An inverted U tube is physically equivalent to an inverted cylinder open at the bottom.

It is useful, when considering the behaviour of fluids in hydrocaptive systems, to take into account that "gauge" pressures are commonly referred to as "negative", but that they are in fact either greater than or equal to zero (vacuum).

The hydrocaptive plane (H.P.) defines the interface between hydrocaptive and non-hydrocaptive elements within a system. At this plane, fluid will not exit the hydrocaptive element even if it is inverted and opened to the atmosphere. Also at this plane, a change in the magnitude of the gravitational force vector will not result in a change in fluid pressure. Of note, the complete submergence of any of these elements in a fluid of equal density to the contained fluid will obliterate air-fluid interfaces and result in transmural pressures at all points being zero in an open container and elastic recoil pressure (mean systemic pressure, or Pms in Fig. 2) in a closed, compliant, container. This is predicted by and consistent with Pascal's Principle. Similarly, in a weightless environment, hydrocaptivity is changed because of the absence of an effective gravitational vector. Contained fluids will remain in place, subject only to unopposed ambient pressure, unless acted on by a new force, in accordance with Newton's First Law.

The static version of the model (Fig. 9.) predicts responses to gravity, but it also serves as an integrated basis for analyzing cardiac-generated pressures (Fig. 10). The link between static and dynamic states of the circulation has been recognized since at least 1897, when Starling's experiments on heart failure called attention to mean systemic pressure (elastic recoil pressure at cardiac standstill) as the equilibrium point around which dynamic pressures pivot during cardiac activity (45). The role of the static model in clarifying the behaviour of the circulation in altered force environments allows the dynamic model to proceed with the effects of gravity already taken into account.

Circulatory Response to +Gz Acceleration

Centrifuge experiments were originally designed to study the physiologic limitations of aviation, not to test rival models of the circulation. Nonetheless, they have provided a wealth of data that may be used for that purpose (50, 51). The demands of piloting aircraft that can sustain higher G forces than the pilots inside provided a practical incentive to discover remedies for what is now termed "acceleration induced loss of consciousness" (GLOC). To that end, both military and civilian centrifuges were built around the time of the Second World War and many of the investigators themselves became experimental human subjects in the successful effort to define and eventually extend the human limits to acceleration (see Wood, 1987)(51).

G-forces in a head-to-foot (+Gz) direction above +4-5 Gz result in GLOC. The use of straining maneuvers and anti-G suits raise that threshold, but at sufficient acceleration, cerebral blood flow becomes critically limited and neurologic sequelae follow. In order, this includes loss of peripheral vision, loss of central vision, then loss of consciousness (51).

Hemodynamic data from centrifuge experiments provide an explicit test of the model presented here. The presence and location of a hydrocaptive plane and the inclusion of the cerebral circulation as a hydrocaptive element can be assessed by examining arterial pressure as a function of both vertical position and G-force. If the systemic circulation behaves as an opposed pair of hydrocaptive elements joined at an H.P. at heart level, as proposed in this model, then increasing +Gz should reveal a constant pressure at heart level, but a decreasing pressure moving cephalad and an increasing pressure moving toward the feet away from the H.P. In contrast, if the circulation behaves as an open container with the heart performing work to elevate blood above it, then the H.P. should occur at head level, and pressures below head level should increase in linear proportion to decreasing height and to increasing +Gz (4). These two alternatives are represented in the upper panels of Fig. 5, which, for clarity, and as a hydrostatic model, excludes cardiac-generated pressures. The combined data from over 60 years of centrifuge experiments in both humans and animals conforms to the hydrocaptive model, but not to the open model.

In retrospect, one of the first and clearest demonstrations of a heart-level H.P. and hydrocaptivity can be seen in the experiments of Brown, Wood, and Lambert in 1949, where the autonomic (baroreceptor) response to acceleration was blocked by tetraethyl ammonium chloride (7). During acceleration to greater than +4 Gz, a marked fall in arterial pressure occurs at head level, with little or no change in arterial pressure at heart level. Additional human centrifuge data reported by Wood, without autonomic blockade, but taken during the first few seconds of +Gz challenge before baroreceptor reflexes can respond, confirm the same hemodynamic pattern (50). Similarly, in more recent experiments with passive head-up tilting (HUT) in humans, Sheriff and Toska detected a divergence between head and heart level blood pressure, with significant decreases in head-level pressure but only a minor change at heart level prior to the onset of autonomic reflexes (44). The same indifference of heart level arterial pressure to HUT was present in dogs with autonomic blockade (43). An open model of the circulation does not predict the observed pattern of responses to acceleration between heart and head-level pressures. Stated another way, if the circulation behaved as an open system and the heart did perform work against gravity to elevate the blood to the head, then the increased weight of the column of blood between heart and head should be evident at increased +Gz. This does not happen. In contrast, the model presented here, with a H.P. occurring at heart level and the cerebral circulation considered as an inverted hydrocaptive element, predicts the response seen in Wood et al.'s experiments.

Rushmer's centrifuge data from 1947 confirm the existence of a cerebral hydrocaptive element as well as a H.P. at heart level on the venous side (41). Because his experiments were performed in animals, he was able to cannulate the cerebral venous sinuses prior to centrifuge runs. The data show subatmospheric pressure in the cerebral sinuses and intracranial cerebrospinal fluid, as well as a proportionate fall in sinus pressure as +Gz acceleration increased. This is also consistent with the hydrocaptive model but not with an open model. The existence of an H.P. at heart level is evident from Rushmer's data when the reference height (h) is calculated from the formula $P = \rho g h$, with pressure measured directly and with known values for ρ and g. Similar, simultaneous, decreases in head level arterial and venous pressure have been observed by Hill in the upright dog, and by Henry et al. in human subjects exposed to +4.5 Gz (22, 25).

Taken together, this data calls into question the convention of referring to "cerebral perfusion pressure" in the upright position as the gradient between arterial pressure measured at the head and intracranial pressure (CSF pressure), while neglecting the immediate downstream cerebral venous pressure. The latter is subatmospheric and in continuity with the arterial blood; and should, therefore, be taken into account as part of the relevant perfusion pressure gradient. When measured carefully, as in Rushmer's experiments, CSF pressure matched cerebral venous pressure, so the gradient Pa – Pcsf is identical to Pa – Pv (all measured at head level). In the absence of direct and simultaneous measurements of all three parameters at head level, the gradient Pa – Pv (both measured at heart level; and usually represented as mean arterial pressure "MAP" and right atrial, or central venous, pressure "CVP") will yield the same perfusion pressure gradient, and with simpler methodology. The concept of including a calculated or inferred cerebral "critical closing pressure", or "zero flow pressure" as the relevant downstream pressure for cerebral perfusion is discussed below.

Recent mathematical modeling by van Heusden, Gisolf and colleagues predicts the empiric results of Sheriff that demonstrate a small but consistent decrease in right atrial pressure with rapid HUT (43, 47). This decrease is in accord with the present model's prediction of a minor decrease in mean systemic pressure (Pms) with the onset of +Gz acceleration or HUT secondary to a translocation of blood from a less compliant jugular venous system to a more compliant lower extremity and abdominal venous capacitance (Fig. 4). In 1895, Hill conducted extensive experiments with abdominal compression in animals, and noted that their ability to compensate for upright positioning was greater with compression (25). This has served as the basis for anti-gravity compression suits ("G-suits") in military aviation, and is viewed in the present model as an increase in P_{ms} (50)

In 1989, Wood summarized the empiric relationship between arterial blood pressure measured at heart level vs. head level as a function of acceleration (from +1 to +6 Gz) with the following formula (53):

$$(P_{heart} - P_{head})/Gz = constant$$

He went on to state that "a magnification of the heart to head level hydrostatic gradient, as opposed to decreases in arterial pressure at heart level, is the major determination of the cephalic hypotension produced by Gz acceleration" (53). Wood , with the assistance of Helmholtz, depicted this "magnification" in a figure demonstrating the +Gz-induced expansion of pressure in a negative direction above the heart, and in a positive direction below it, with pressure at heart level remaining constant (52). Neither Wood nor other aviation physiologists elaborated a new conceptual model of the circulation based on this observation, however.

A caveat that is inherent to the studies cited above is that measurement of arterial pressures was performed from radial or upper extremity digital sites – either elevated to head level or remaining at heart level. While it is fair to assume that the arteries of the upper extremity act as physical extensions of the pressure transduction system, and therefore, the elevation of the transducer to head level is an adequate estimate of transmural pressure at head level, it should also be affirmed that, by definition, elevating the pressure transducer will generate lower recorded pressures regardless of what is being measured. The reason why data from these studies was not begging the question is that the differential pressure changes between transducers at heart vs. head level in response to changes in +Gz acceleration are an accurate reflection of a real physiologic hydrocaptive plane and a real physiologic hydrocaptive element, respectively. This same pattern of differential responses between heart and level transducers would not arise from interrogation of an open system.

The original hypothesis that the cerebral circulation, contained within a rigid cranium and surrounded by a non-displaceable fluid compartment, was resistant to the effects of +Gz acceleration was proposed by Hill in 1895 and again by Ranke in 1938 and tested more recently by Cirovic and in the present study (9, 25, 39). Ranke developed a conceptual model of the cerebral circulation that distinguished between the blood supply to the brain and to the eye. Since the cerebral vessels are encased within rigid, fluid-filled skull, but the eyes are exposed to atmospheric pressure, Ranke theorized that the eye vessels would respond to negative transmural pressure by collapsing at lower G-forces than the cerebral vessels. This model corresponds to experimental observations as well as to the hydrocaptive model, which predicts subatmospheric pressures in the cerebral circulation that fall in proportion to +Gz acceleration. Ranke's theoretical model was noted by Wood, who understood that subatmospheric pressure in the cerebral venous system could play a role in maintaining cerebral perfusion pressure in the face of +Gz, but these compatible observations were never integrated into a single model of the systemic circulation (49).

It should be borne in mind that humans spend a majority of their lives in the upright position at the equivalent of +1 Gz. It is not surprising, then, that the transition from supine (0 Gz) to upright (+1 Gz) does not result in a significant fall in cerebral blood flow; or more properly stated, that the transition from the normal awake human upright position to supine does not result in a significant increase in cerebral blood flow (1, 33). Even in the dog the transition from supine to head up results in no change in cerebral blood flow in the absence of increased intracranial pressure (13). Only when G-forces are extended to greater than 4-5 G does the transmural pressure in the jugular venous system, and possibly in the arterial system and the accessory vertebral plexus system, decrease enough to cause sufficient vascular collapse and increased vascular resistance to diminish cerebral blood flow (9, 16). There is no need to invoke an open system, along with it's imputation of cardiac work against gravity, to explain decreased cerebral blood flow at extraordinary +Gz values. Increased vascular resistance from vessels, primarily extracranial, that are able to collapse at extraordinary +Gz suffices. This is in addition to the observation that an open system model fails to account for the centrifuge data cited, and that it has not resulted in a tenable anatomical or physiological model. Because of the differential compliance between the jugular veins and the abdominal and lower extremity veins, increased +Gz acceleration will also translocate blood away from the central compartment, and therefore, decrease Pms and with it, cardiac output and arterial pressure. This is also incorporated into the present model (Fig. 9 and Fig. 10).

Hemodynamics of the Giraffe

The most obvious terrestrial test case for theories concerning the role of gravity in the circulation is the giraffe. In 1960, Goetz made direct hemodynamic measurements (17). He noted that the arterial pressure, measured at heart level, was higher than in humans or in other mammals. This led to the hypothesis that the giraffe's heart had to generate extraordinary pressures in order to pump blood an extraordinary distance uphill. Five years later, however, applying the principles of hydraulics first elucidated by Pascal and Bernoulli, Burton commented that, "In the circulation, it is no harder to pump blood uphill than downhill" (8). It has also been noted, with symmetric logic, that giraffes lower their heads to well below heart level while drinking, but that they have not been noted to lower their arterial pressure accordingly (34). As well, by Poiseuille's equation, the perfusion pressure across a cerebral vascular loop that is substantially longer than a human's would be expected to be proportionately higher, without invoking either the need for the giraffe to raise its arterial pressure when its head is up or lower it when its head is down.

More recent measurements were made by Hargens et al. in 1987 (20). They measured both arterial and venous transmural pressures at a variety of elevations within the vascular system. Of note, they recorded venous pressures in the foot that correlated with an expected heart-to-foot hydrostatic gradient. In commenting on the corresponding arterial pressures, they noted that they correlated with an expected head-to-foot hydrostatic gradient. Their data, however, show that the animal is approximately 400 cm tall when standing upright, and the arterial pressures at foot level are 260 mmHg. Because they did not subtract the arterial pressure generated by the left ventricle from the total arterial pressure, they overestimated the hydrostatic (gravitational) gradient of arterial blood. Doing so yields an expected heart-to-foot, not head-to-foot value. Together with their venous pressure measurements and the data of Goetz, which revealed right atrial pressures of approximately atmospheric, these two studies demonstrate a H.P. at heart level, consistent with that depicted in the bottom panels of Fig. 2.

Controversy surrounds the interpretations of direct jugular venous pressure measurements in the giraffe. Hargens et al. noted that the transmural pressures in the jugular vein were less than, and in the opposite direction to, what would be expected from a standing column of blood, or from one limb of a siphon (20). In contrast, Badeer interprets the jugular venous values as consistent with a siphon model (an inverted U tube with equal limbs) once the effects of resistance to viscous flow are taken into account (2). Measurements made in humans have not resolved the conflict. Transmural pressures in the internal jugular vein of upright humans fail to reveal a haemostatic profile consistent with either a standing column of fluid or with a siphon (10).

Germane to this debate is the fact that both humans and giraffes may use non-jugular routes (vertebral venous plexus veins) as the predominant venous return pathway from the elevated head (16, 32). The possibility remains that catheter measurements in partially collapsed internal jugular veins are subject to vessel wall artifact when the catheter tip migrates into and opens a potential space that is not in continuity with the remainder of the fluid column. Any pathway of fluid continuity from cerebral veins to the right atrium is sufficient to establish a gravitationally neutral hydrocaptive element, however, whether it passes through the jugular or the vertebral venous plexus system. To date, there is no data to suggest that a discontinuity exists in the steady-state venous drainage of the upright head in either human or giraffe. Careful measurements of central venous pressure in the anesthetized dog have reconfirmed Guyton's original observation that the pressure in the right atrium is not sensitive to body position (13). What is clear from the data taken from the giraffe by both Goetz and Hargens, is that both arterial and central venous measurements are consistent with the presence of an H.P. at heart level; and therefore, with the central proposition of the hydrocaptive model.

The Absence of a Starling Resistor in the Cerebral Circulation

Originally described by Starling in 1912 and refined by Holt in 1941, a Starling resistor is simply a collapsible fluid-filled conduit surrounded by an external pressure that is lower than inlet pressure, but higher than outlet pressure (27, 46). Descriptively, flow rate through the resistor is a function of the gradient between inlet and intermediate/external pressure rather than the difference between inlet and outlet pressure (11, 12, 29, 30, 37, 38, 48). As pointed out by Badeer and Hicks, however, confirmation of this has been less than clear (3). For example, one report of experimental evidence for the existence of a cerebral Starling resistor itself demonstrates a propagation of venous pressure waves retrograde from internal jugular to cerebral veins (29). Similarly, in the upright position in both human and animal studies, cerebral venous pressures are subatmospheric, reflecting the enclosed conduit of blood connecting them to the right atrium (22, 25, 40). These observations are incompatible with Permutt's description of a "vascular waterfall", where pressure at the Starling resistor element is assumed to be insulated from downstream pressure changes (37, 38).

Regardless of the state of experimental confirmation for physical models, the application of the Starling resistor concept to the cerebral circulation in particular is problematic (15, 24, 34). This is because, however collapsible, the intracranial vessels are surrounded by an incompressible fluid medium which is in turn encased in a rigid skull. For intracranial vessels to collapse, their volume loss has to be displaced, but there is no sufficiently expansible medium within the skull to displace it (9, 25).

Prior to the model of Cirovic, all previous models of Starling resistors have contained elements around the intermediate portion of the conduit that are displaceable, thus allowing collapse of the conduit (27, 37, 46). Cirovic, using a rigidly encased fluid medium that better simulates the cranium, demonstrated that collapsible conduit within a simulated fluid and cranium model sustains flow and remains distended to its original volume even when draining into a low pressure outlet (9). The model presented in Fig. 3, with data in Table 1, demonstrates the same result, but with the added feature of maintaining fluid flow through a subatmospheric inverted U tube, and through collapsible conduit simulating extracranial jugular veins.

Together with the model of Hicks and Badeer, this data confirms that collapsible but non-collapsed intracranial vessels, along with partially collapsed extracranial vessels, are capable of maintaining fluid continuity and siphon flow even without a positive pressure source. Data indicating that the human cerebral venous return shifts from predominantly jugular to predominantly vertebral plexus drainage during the transition from supine to upright positioning does not change the physiology qualitatively (16). The cerebral circulation, like all systemic vascular loops, has its inlet and outlet at the same vertical level, so no active siphoning effect will occur in vivo. The point of establishing siphon flow was to test, and reject, the hypothesis that intracranial pressure constitutes an intermediate Starling resistor pressure that should be counted as the relevant downstream pressure for cerebral perfusion. Data from Rushmer confirm that cerebrospinal fluid pressure at the level of the cranium mirrors intracranial venous pressure at all +Gz forces tested (40). This is consistent with the model presented here, as well as with the model of Cirovic (9).

Seymour et al. have raised a different objection to the application of siphon principles to the cerebral circulation (42). They argue that the partially collapsed state of the jugular vessels increases viscous resistance to flow so that the potential energy of venous blood as it flows down to the right atrium is lost to resistive heat loss, and is therefore unavailable to aid in the ascent of the arterial column of blood. The physical model presented in Fig. 3 demonstrates that the "arterial" column of fluid is, in fact, sustained by the partially collapsed "venous" column of fluid – otherwise, siphon flow, driven by a differential height between the upstream and downstream baths, could not occur through the system in the absence of a positive pressure source. Even if all cerebral venous return was confined to the partially collapsed jugular veins, rather than more rigidly supported extra-jugular vessels, the energetic implications remain the same: the heart works against resistance, not against gravity.

It is also important to distinguish between static and dynamic effects of gravity on the circulation. There is no doubt that a partially collapsed jugular vein will present an increased resistance to flow, but as long as fluid continuity is maintained, the hydrostatic pressure of the arterial column will be matched by its venous return limb, regardless of any difference in diameter. As a consequence, the heart will only be required to work against viscous flow resistance, not against gravity. The observation that the human cerebral circulation sustains approximately 750 mL/min of blood flow in the normal upright human position suggests that, as in this model and the model of Hicks and Badeer, venous fluid continuity is maintained despite a tendency of the jugular element to collapse (3, 23). This has also been confirmed by MRI imaging of cerebral blood flow and cerebral tissue compartments as well as by ultrasound insonation of the cerebral straight sinus in both supine and upright positions (1, 33).

The Dynamic Model

Following the concept of Levy (28, 36), as the heart begins to beat from a state of circulatory arrest, arterial pressures rise above Pms and venous pressures fall below P_{ms} (Fig. 10A). This coincides with a translocation of blood from the veins into the arteries (Fig. 10C). Arterial pressure (Pa) is the sum of P_{ms} and left ventricular derived pressure (P_{LVD}), some of which contributes to a kinetic component ($1/2 \rho u2$), and the remainder to lateral pressure. Similarly, venous pressure (Pv) is the result of right ventricular suction (PRVS) reducing P_{ms}. Right atrial pressure (PRA) is simply a local distortion of mean systemic pressure caused by the action of the right heart.

Because this model predicts subatmospheric pressure in the elevated cerebral veins and sinuses, it also has utility for explaining several clinical observations, including: 1) an explanation for venous air embolism (VAE) in both spontaneously breathing and mechanically ventilated patients undergoing surgery in the upright position; and 2) an explanation for why the tendency to VAE increases as the site of surgical venous perforation is elevated higher than the heart (24, 34). In the absence of a model that incorporates the mechanics of siphons (here referred to as hydrocaptive elements), the phenomenon of VAE and the proportion between the tendency to VAE and elevation of the surgical perforation above the heart remains unexplained. Similarly, the observation of subatmospheric venous and sagittal sinus pressures in mechanically ventilated subjects remains unexplained in the absence of the principle of the siphon (hydrocaptivity). In addition, the model presented here correctly predicts: 3) the existence of a hydrocaptive plane in mammals at heart level, rather than head level; and 4) the differential hemodynamic response of cerebral versus lower extremity vascular circuits to increased +Gz forces.

References

1. Alperin N, Lee S, Sivaramakrishnan A, and Hushek S. Quantifying the effect of posture on intracranial physiology in humans by MRI flow studies. J Magn Reson Imaging 22: 591-596, 2005.

2. Badeer H. Haemodynamics of the jugular vein in the giraffe. Nature 332: 788-789, 1988.

3. Badeer H and Hicks J. Hemodynamics of vascular 'waterfall': is the analogy justified? Respir Physiol 87: 205-217, 1992.

4. Banks R, Brinkley J, Allnutt R, and Harding R. Human Response to Acceleration. In: Fundamentals of Aerospace Medicine (4th ed.), edited by Davis J, Stepanek J, Johnson R and Fogarty J. Philadelphia: Wolters Kluwer Lippincott Williams & Wilkins, 2008.

5. Beard DA and Feigl EO. Understanding Guyton's venous return curves. Am J Physiol Heart Circ Physiol 301: H629-633, 2011.

6. Brengelmann GL. A critical analysis of the view that right atrial pressure determines venous return. J Appl Physiol 94: 849-859, 2003.

7. Brown GJ, Wood E, and Lambert E. Effects of tetra-ethyl-ammonium chloride on the cardiovascular reactions in man to changes in posture and exposure to centrifugal force. J Appl Physiol 2: 117-132, 1949.

8. Burton A. Physiology and Biophysics of the Circulation. Chicago: Year Book Medical Publishers, 1965.

9. Cirovic S, Walsh C, and Fraser W. A mechanical model of cerebral circulation during sustained acceleration. Aviat Space Environ Med 72: 704-712, 2001.

10. Dawson E, Secher N, Dalsgaard M, Ogoh S, Yoshiga C, González-Alonso J, Steensberg A, and Raven P. Standing up to the challenge of standing: a siphon does not support cerebral blood flow in humans. Am J Physiol Regul Integr Comp Physiol 287: R911-914, 2004.

11. Dewey R, Pieper H, and Hunt W. Experimental cerebral hemodynamics. Vasomotor tone, critical closing pressure, and vascular bed resistance. J Neurosurg 41: 597-606, 1974.

12. Early C, Dewey R, Pieper H, and Hunt W. Dynamic pressure-flow relationships of brain blood flow in the monkey. J Neurosurg 41: 590-596, 1974.

13. Ernst P, Albin M, and Bunegin L. Intracranial and spinal cord hemodynamics in the sitting position in dogs in the presence and absence of increased intracranial pressure. Anesth Analg 70: 147-153, 1990.

14. Fishman A and Richards D. Circulation of the Blood: Men and Ideas. Bethesda, MD: American Physiological Society, 1982.

15. Gisolf J, Gisolf A, van Lieshout J, and Karemaker J. The siphon controversy: an integration of concepts and the brain as baffle. Am J Physiol Regul Integr Comp Physiol 289: R627-629, 2005.

16. Gisolf J, van Lieshout J, van Heusden K, Pott F, Stok W, and Karemaker J. Human cerebral venous outflow pathway depends on posture and central venous pressure. J Physiol 560: 317-327, 2004.

17. Goetz R, Warren J, Gauer O, Patterson J, Doyle J, Keen E, and McGregor M. Circulation of the Giraffe. Circulation Research 8: 1049-1058, 1960.

18. Guyton A and Greganti F. A physiologic reference point for measuring circulatory pressures in the dog; particularly venous pressure. Am J Physiol 185: 137-141, 1956.

19. Hammond N. The Cambridge Companion to Pascal. Cambridge: Cambridge University Press, 2003.

20. Hargens A, Millard R, Pettersson K, and Johansen K. Gravitational haemodynamics and oedema prevention in the giraffe. Nature 329: 59-60, 1987.

21. Harvey W. Anatomical Studies on the Motion of The Heart and Blood, 1628.

22. Henry J, Gauer O, Kety S, and Kramer K. Factors maintaining cerebral circulation during gravitational stress. J Clin Invest 30: 292-300, 1951.

23.   Hicks J and Badeer H. Siphon mechanism in collapsible tubes: application to circulation of the giraffe head. Am J Physiol 256: R567-571, 1989.

24.   Hicks J and Munis J. The siphon controversy counterpoint: the brain need not be "baffling". Am J Physiol Regul Integr Comp Physiol 289: R629-632, 2005.

25.   Hill L. The influence of the force of gravity on the circulation of the blood. J Physiol 15: 18-53, 1895.

26.   Hinghofer-Szalkay H. Gravity, the hydrostatic indifference concept and the cardiovascular system. Eur J Appl Physiol 111: 163-174, 2011.

27.   Holt JP. The collapse factor in the measurement of venous pressure: the flow of fluid through collapsible tubes. Am J Physiol 134: 292-299, 1941.

28.   Levy M. The cardiac and vascular factors that determine systemic blood flow. Circ Res 44: 739-747, 1979.

29.   Luce J, Huseby J, Kirk W, and Butler J. A Starling resistor regulates cerebral venous outflow in dogs. J Appl Physiol 53: 1496-1503, 1982.

30.   Magder S. Starling resistor versus compliance. Which explains the zero-flow pressure of a dynamic arterial pressure-flow relation? Circ Res 67: 209-220, 1990.

31.   McCarthy EL. Mariotte's Bottle. Science 80: 100, 1934.

32.   Mitchell G, Bobbitt J, and Devries S. Cerebral perfusion pressure in giraffe: modelling the effects of head-raising and -lowering. J Theor Biol 252: 98-108, 2008.

33.   Mosso M, Schmid-Priscoveanu A, Straumann D, and Baumgartner R. Absence of gravity-dependent modulation of straight sinus flow velocity in healthy humans. Ultrasound Med Biol 34: 726-729, 2008.

34.   Munis J and Lozada L. Giraffes, siphons, and starling resistors. Cerebral perfusion pressure revisited. J Neurosurg Anesthesiol 12: 290-296, 2000.

35. Munis JR. Letter to the editor: "A return to the venous return controversy: a visual aid for combatants". Am J Physiol Heart Circ Physiol 304: H487-488, 2013.

36. Munis JR, Bhatia S, and Lozada LJ. Peripheral venous pressure as a hemodynamic variable in neurosurgical patients. Anesth Analg 92: 172-179, 2001.

37. Permutt S, Bromberger-Barnea B, and Bane H. Alveolar pressure, pulmonary venous pressure, and the vascular waterfall. Med Thorac 19: 239-260, 1962.

38. Permutt S and Riley R. Hemodynamics of collapsible vessels with tone: the vascular waterfall. J Appl Physiol 18: 924-932, 1963.

39. Ranke O. The effect of acceleration [in German]. Luftfahrtmedizin 2: 243-258, 1938.

40. Rushmer R. A roentgenographic study of the effect of a pneumatic anti-blackout suit on the hydrostatic columns in man exposed to positive radial acceleration. Am J Physiol 151: 459-468, 1947.

41. Rushmer R, Beckman E, and Lee D. Protection of the cerebral circulation by the cerebrospinal fluid under the influence of radial acceleration. Am J Physiol 151: 355-365, 1947.

42. Seymour R, Hargens A, and Pedley T. The heart works against gravity. Am J Physiol 265: R715-720, 1993.

43. Sheriff D. Hypotensive effect of push-pull gravitational stress occurs after autonomic blockade. J Appl Physiol 95: 167-171, 2003.

44. Sheriff D, Inger-Helene N, and Toska K. Hemodynamic consequences of rapid changes in posture in humans. J Appl Physiol 103: 452-458, 2007.

45. Starling E. The Arris and Gale Lectures on some points in the pathology of heart disease; Lecture II. The effects of heart failure on the circulation. Lancet 1: 652-655, 1897.

46. Starling E. Principles Of Human Physiology. Philadelphia: Lea & Febiger, 1912.

47. van Heusden K, Gisolf J, Stok W, Dijkstra S, and Karemaker J. Mathematical modeling of gravitational effects on the circulation: importance of the time course of venous pooling and blood volume changes in the lungs. Am J Physiol Heart Circ Physiol 291: H2152-2165, 2006.

48. West J, Dollery C, and Naimark A. Distribution of blood flow in isolated lung; relation to vascular and alveolar pressures. J Appl Physiol 19: 713-724, 1964.

49. Wood E. Hydrostatic homeostatic effects during changing force environments. Aviat Space Environ Med 61: 366-373, 1990.

50. Wood E. Prevention of +Gz-induced loss of consciousness. Aviat Space Environ Med 63: 226-227, 1992.

51. Wood E. Some effects of the force environment on the heart, lungs and circulation. Clin Invest Med 10: 401-427, 1987.

52. Wood E and Lindberg E. Acceleration. In: Physiology of Man in Space, edited by Brown J. New York: Academic Press, 1963, p. 63-85.

53. Wood E and Sturm R. Human centrifuge non-invasive measurements of arterial pressure at eye level during Gz acceleration. Aviat Space Environ Med 60: 1005-1010, 1989.

www.ingramcontent.com/pod-product-compliance
Lightning Source LLC
Chambersburg PA
CBHW041257180526
45172CB00003B/879